YOUR KNOWLEDGE HAS VALUE

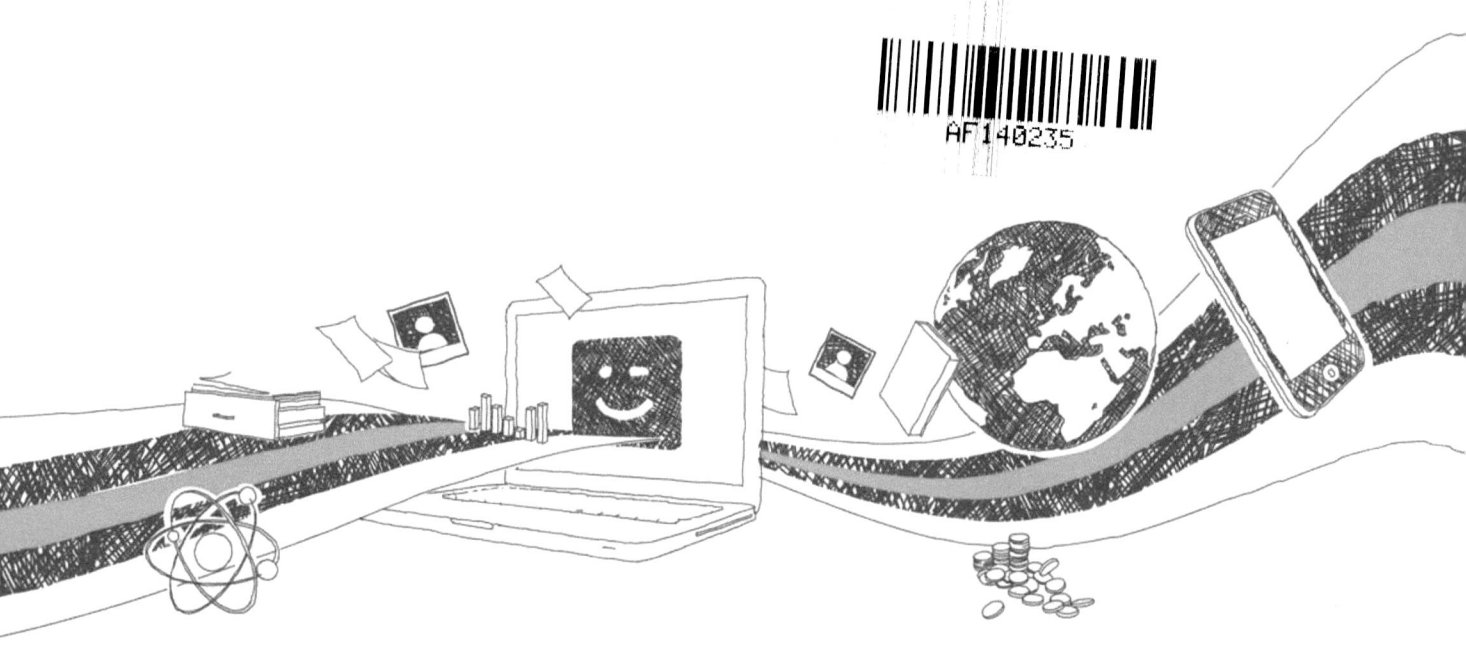
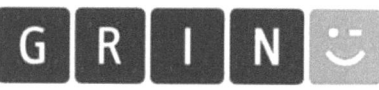

Bibliographic information published by the German National Library:

The German National Library lists this publication in the National Bibliography; detailed bibliographic data are available on the Internet at http://dnb.dnb.de .

Imprint:

Copyright © 2018 GRIN Verlag
Print and binding: Books on Demand GmbH, Norderstedt Germany
ISBN: 9783668694637

This book at GRIN:

https://www.grin.com/document/423950

Sagar Pamu

Tuberculosis and its Advanced Therapy

GRIN Verlag

GRIN - Your knowledge has value

Since its foundation in 1998, GRIN has specialized in publishing academic texts by students, college teachers and other academics as e-book and printed book. The website www.grin.com is an ideal platform for presenting term papers, final papers, scientific essays, dissertations and specialist books.

Visit us on the internet:

http://www.grin.com/

http://www.facebook.com/grincom

http://www.twitter.com/grin_com

Tuberculosis and its Advanced Therapy

Author

Sagar Pamu

List of Contents

TUBERCULOSIS AND ITS ADVANCED THERAPY

1. Introduction

Tuberculosis [TB] is an infectious disease that can affect any part of the body, mainly an infection of the lungs.

In Neo-Latin word, tuberculosis is termed as 'TUBERCLE' which means round nodule and 'OSIS' which means condition.

The causative organism for tuberculosis is Mycobacterium tuberculosis in human and Mycobacterium bovis in animals. Mycobacterium tuberculosis is small, aerobic, nonmotile bacillus [1]. The other causative organisms are Mycobacterium africanum and Mycobacterium microti. The non-mycobacterium genuses are Mycobacterium leprae, Mycobacterium avium, Mycobacterium asiaticum. The M.Tuberculosis complex consists of M.africanum, M.bovis, M.canetti, and M.microti.

CLASSIFICATION

Figure No-1: Classification of Tuberculosis [2]

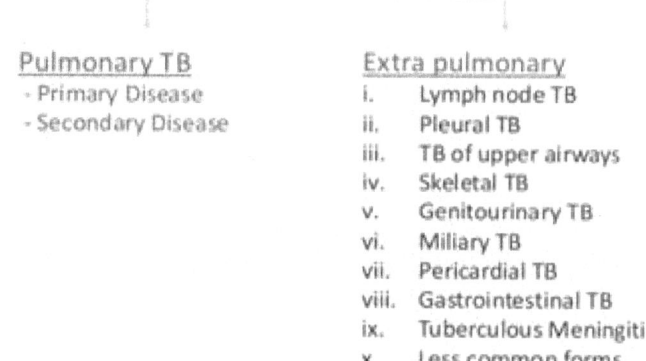

Pulmonary TB	Extra pulmonary	
- Primary Disease	i.	Lymph node TB
- Secondary Disease	ii.	Pleural TB
	iii.	TB of upper airways
	iv.	Skeletal TB
	v.	Genitourinary TB
	vi.	Miliary TB
	vii.	Pericardial TB
	viii.	Gastrointestinal TB
	ix.	Tuberculous Meningitis
	x.	Less common forms

2. Epidemiology

According to WORLD HEALTH ORGANISATION (WHO), in 2012 they estimated around 8.6 million cases in which women were found approximately around 2.9. Most cases were found in Africa (27%) and Asia (58%), with a highest incidence in India (2.0-2.4 million), China (0.9-1.1 million); and total accounted the number of cases is 38% [3].

The incidence rate of TB was eventually declined from 1997-2001 but increased in 2001 due to more number of HIV infected patient's cases in Africa. Later there was a reduction of 1.3% per year since 2002. The absolute numbers of cases were also decreasing, but this has begun in 2006.

The estimated prevalent cases in 2012 were around 12 million, corresponding to 169 cases per one lakh population [3]. TB prevalence is declining from the early 1990's (before incidence started to decline). This is largely due to the introduction of DOTS strategy, which may have contributed to the reduction of chronic and cases which are untreated and duration of illness.

In 2012 TB mortality cases are estimated to be 1.3 million deaths including 320000 HIV associated cases. Since 1990 a drop of 45% TB mortality rate has been observed [4].

Figure No.2: Incidence, prevalence, and mortality of TB [4]

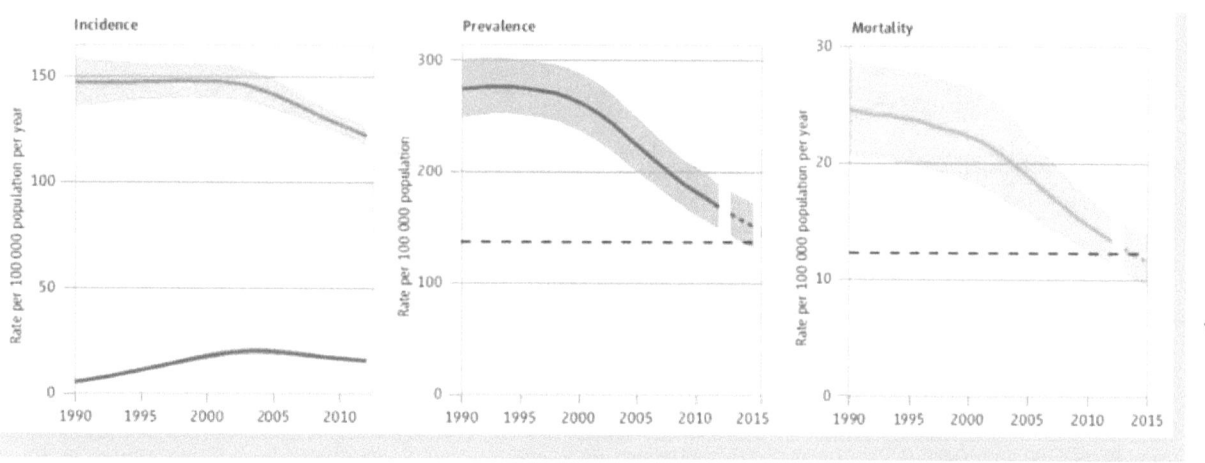

The spread of tuberculosis can happen while coughing without covering mouth, crowded places with poor ventilation, spitting everywhere. From the area of damaged tissue, TB bacteria enter into the bloodstream which spreads throughout the body, set up many foci of infection; all appears tiny and white tubercles in the tissues [5].

Most important risk factor globally is HIV; 13% of people with TB are infected by the virus [6]. Chronic lung disease (CLD) is one of the risk factors. Silicosis increases the risk about 30-folds [7]. Cigarette smokers have nearly twice the risk of TB compared to nonsmokers [8].People with prolonged, frequent, or close contact with people with TB are at particularly high risk of becoming infected, with an estimated 22% infection rate [9].

The severe symptoms are a Persistent cough, Chest pain, Coughing with bloody sputum, Shortness of breath, Urine discoloration, Cloudy and reddish urine, Fever with chills and Fatigue.

3. Pathogenesis

Figure No-3: Pathogenesis of TB [10]

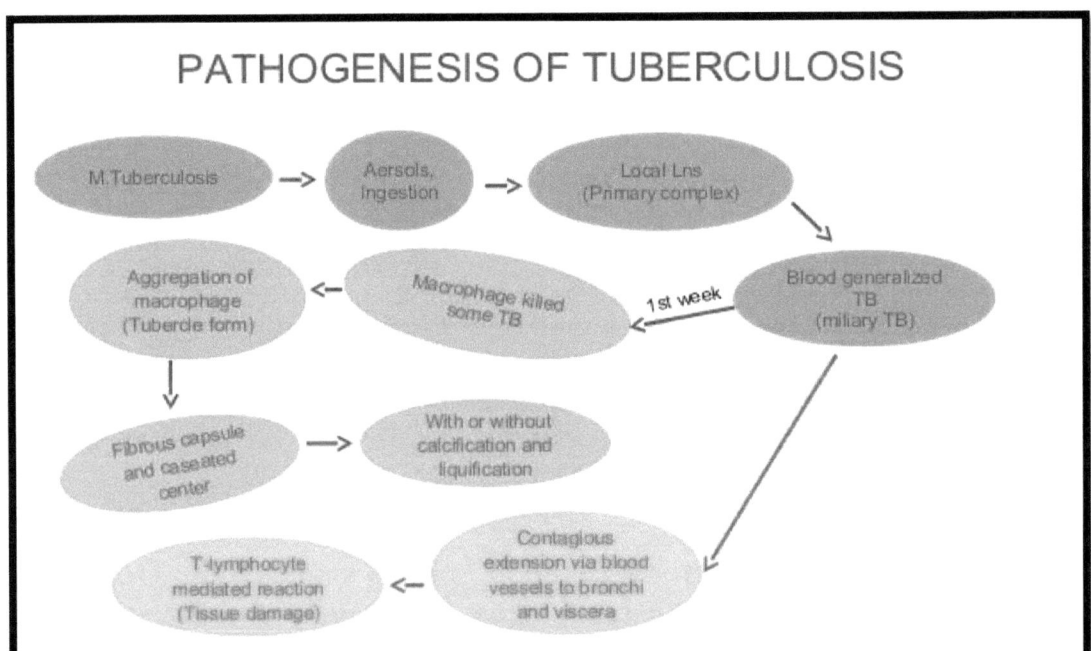

4. Types of Tuberculosis

A. **Pulmonary TB**: If tuberculosis infection becomes active, it most commonly involves the lungs (about 90% of cases) [11, 12].

There are two types of pulmonary TB, one is **Primary TB** where the infection vary from inter-individual conditions and it applies who has not been infected formerly or immunized and another is **Secondary TB** where it doesn't varies from inter-individual but it applies who has already been infected formerly.

B. **Extrapulmonary TB**: Around 15–20% of active cases, the infection spreads outside the lungs, causing other kinds of TB [13]. These collectively termed as "extrapulmonary tuberculosis" [14].

There are 10 different types of extra pulmonary TB; they are

Lymph Node TB which is frequently seen in HIV infected patients with symptoms like swelling of lymph nodes commonly at cervical and supracervical.

Pleural TB which has involvement of pleura and penetration of tubercle bacilli into pleural space.

TB of Upper Airways involves larynx, pharynx, and epiglottis with symptoms like dysphasia and chronic productive cough.

Genitourinary TB occurs in the genitourinary tract with symptoms like urinary frequency, dysuria, and hematuria.

Skeletal TB involves the parts like spine, hip and knee with symptoms like pain in hip joints and knees, swelling of knees and trauma.

Gastrointestinal TB involves part of GI tract with symptoms like abdominal pain, diarrhea, and weight loss.

TB Meningitis and Tuberculoma which results from the spread of primary and secondary TB.

TB Pericarditis in which 1-8% of all TB cases spreads mainly from mediastinal or hilar nodes or from lungs.

Military Or Disseminated TB is producing lesions at different extrapulmonary sites due to the entry of infection into the pulmonary veins. "Disseminated Tuberculosis" is the most serious and widespread form of TB, which is also known as miliary tuberculosis [15]. About 10% of extra pulmonary cases include military TB [16].

Less Common Forms includes uveitis, panopthalmitis and painful hypersensitivity related phlyetenular conjunctivitis.

5. Diagnosis

1. **Bacteriological test:-**

   a) Zeihl – Nielsen stain

   b) Auramine stain (fluorescence microscopy)

2. **Sputum culture test:-**

   a) Lowenstein – Jensen solid medium – 4-18wks

   b) Liquid medium – 8-14days

   c) Agar medium – 7-14days

3. **Radiography :-** Chest x-ray [CXR]

4. **Nucleic acid amplification:-**

   Species identification, several hours, Low sensitivity, high cost, most useful for the confirmation of tuberculosis in persons with AFB positive sputa

5. **Tuberculin Skin Test:-**

   Injection into the skin of the lower arm

   48-72 hours later checked for reaction

   Diagnosis is done based on the size of the wheel

   Dose = 0.1ml contains 0.04ug tuberculin PPD

   Less than 6mm – negative

6mm or greater but less than 15mm – hypersensitive to tuberculin protein, may be due to previous TB infection, BCG or exposure to atypical mycobacterium

>= 15mm – strongly hypersensitive to tuberculin protein, suggestive of TB infection or disease

6. Other Biological Examinations:-

Cell count (lymphocytes)

Protein (pandy and Rivalta tests) – ascites, meningitis and pleural effusion

Chest X-ray and sputum cultures for acid-fast bacilli are part of the initial evaluation [17]. Nucleic acid amplification and adenosine deaminase testing may allow rapid diagnosis of TB [18]. In Sarcoidosis, Hodgkin's lymphoma, malnutrition, and active tuberculosis the test may be falsely negative [19].

Prevention and control efforts of tuberculosis majorly depend on the infant's vaccination, an exact diagnosis and appropriate treatment of active cases [20]. The preventive measures are you should keep mask to avoid exposure and take BCG vaccine prior and for regular medical follow up, BCG vaccine in children decreases the risk of the infection by 20% and the risk of infection turning into disease by 60% [21].Isolation of patient is necessary so that others will not get affected, ventilation is necessary never be in a dark room mostly natural sunlight is better, use UV germicidal irradiation.

6. Management of Tuberculosis

First Line Drugs –

- Isoniazid
- Rifampicin
- Ethambutol
- Pyrazinamide
- Streptomycin

Second Line Drugs –

- Ethionamide
- Levofloxacin
- Moxifloxacin
- Capreomycin
- Cycloserine
- Kanamycin
- Amikacin

7. Treatment Duration and comments

Table No-1: Treatment Duration and comments for Tuberculosis [22]

Intensive therapy	Continuation therapy	Comments
2 months of HRZE	4 months of HR	----
2 months of HRZE	4 months of HRE	This is only for new TB patients with high levels of isoniazid resistance, and where drug susceptibility testing is not done in new patients or results are unavailable before the continuation phase begins

8. Isoniazid

Group – Anti mycobacterial agent

Tablet – 100mg, 300mg

Injection – 25mg/ml in 2ml ampoule

MOA – It is a prodrug and must be activated by the enzyme KatG [23]. This catalyzes the formation of an isonicotinic acyl radical thereby couples with the NADH to form nicotinoyl-NAD. This complex will tightly bind to the carrier protein reductase InhA, thereby blocks the action of fatty acid synthase. This process will inhibit the mycolic acid synthesis. Isoniazid is a monoamine oxidase inhibitor[24].

Figure No-4: Mechanism of action of Isoniazid

Pharmacokinetic Data: Isoniazid absorbs rapidly and readily diffuses into all fluids and tissues. The plasma half-life varies from less than one hour in fast acetylators to more than three hours in slow acetylators. It is largely excreted in the urine within 24hrs, mostly as inactive metabolites.

Routes of Administration: Oral, Intramuscular, Intravenous

Pregnancy Category: C

Dosage and Administration:-

Adults and children – 5mg/kg (4-6mg/kg) daily, max 300mg

10mg/kg three times weekly

15mg/kg two times weekly

Preventive Therapy:-

Adults – 300mg/kg daily for six months at least

Children – 5mg/kg daily (max 300mg) for six months at least

Contraindications: - Hypersensitivity which is known and hepatic disease which is active

Adverse Effects:-

Isoniazid is generally well tolerated at recommended doses. Hypersensitivity reactions occasionally occur during the first weeks of treatment.

The risk of peripheral neuropathy is excluded if vulnerable patients receive daily supplements of pyridoxine. Neurological disturbances include convulsions, optic neuritis which can develop in susceptible individuals at later stages of treatment. Withdrawal of isoniazid occasionally is necessary.

Hepatitis is an uncommon but potentially serious reaction that can usually be averted by the prompt withdrawal of treatment. More often, however, a sharp rise in serum concentrations of hepatic transaminases at the outset of treatment is not of clinical significance and usually resolves spontaneously during the continuation of treatment.

Drug Interactions: - Isoniazid tends to raise plasma concentrations of phenytoin and carbamazepine by inhibiting their metabolism in the liver. The absorption of isoniazid is impaired by aluminum hydroxide.

Over Dosage: - Nausea, vomiting, dizziness, blurred vision and slurring of speech occurs within 30minutes to three hours of overdosage. Coma may occur followed by respiratory depression and a state of unconsciousness can due to by massive poisoning. Severe intractable seizures may occur. Emesis and gastric lavage can be of value within a few hours of ingestion. Subsequently, hemodialysis may be of value. Administration of high doses of pyridoxine is necessary to prevent peripheral neuritis.

Storage: - Tablets should be kept in well-closed container, protected from light. The injection solution should be stored in ampoules protected from light

9. Rifampicin

Group – Antimycobacterial agent

Capsule or Tablet – 150mg, 300mg, 450mg, 600mg

MOA - Rifampicin inhibits bacterial DNA-dependent RNA synthesis by binding to the pocket of the RNA polymerase β subunit within the DNA/RNA channel [25]. The drug prevents RNA synthesis by blocking elongation and preventing synthesis of host bacterial proteins.

Pharmacokinetics – Rifampicin is orally administered which results in peak plasma concentrations in about two to four hours. It gets easily absorbed from GI tract and only 7% of the drug excreted unchanged in urine, 60-65% is excreted in feces.

Routes of Administration – Oral, IV

Pregnancy Category – C

Dosage and Administration:-

Adults and children – 10mg/kg (8-12mg/kg) daily, max 600mg daily, two or three times weekly

Contraindications:-

Known hypersensitivity to rifampicin and Hepatic dysfunction

Side Effects:-

Common side effects are nausea, vomiting, diarrhea, and loss of appetite [26]; it often turns urine, sweat, and tears a red or orange color [26]. Liver problems like hepatitis, toxicity may occur. It is part of the treatment of active tuberculosis during pregnancy, even though its safety in pregnancy is not known [26].

Adverse Effects:-

In most of the patients it is well tolerated at recommended doses, was gastrointestinal tolerance can be severe. With intermittent administration skin rashes, fever, thrombocytopenia is most likely to occur. In HIV positive TB patient's exfoliative dermatitis is more frequent. Temporary oliguria, dyspnea, and hemolytic anemia have also been reported in patients taking the drug 3 times weekly. These reactions generally occur if the regimen is changed to one with daily dosage. There is a moderate rise in serum concentration of bilirubin and transaminases. However, dose-related hepatitis can occur which is potentially fatal. It is consequently important not to exceed the maximum recommended daily dose of 10mg/kg (600mg)

Drug Interactions:-

Rifampicin-induced hepatic enzymes; drugs metabolized in the liver may increase the dosage requirements. These include oral anticoagulants, phenytoin, cimetidine, cyclosporine, corticosteroids, steroid contraceptives, oral hypoglycemic agents and digitalis glycosides. Since rifampicin reduces the effectiveness of the oral contraceptive pill, women should consequently be advised to choose alternative options for contraception.

Over Dosage:-

Gastric lavage can be done if undertaken within a few hours of ingestion. The Central nervous function may depress with very large doses. For rifampicin toxicity, there is no specific antidote for but the treatment is supportive.

Storage:-

Capsules and tablets should be stored in tightly closed containers which it is to protect from light.

10. Pyrazinamide

Group- Antimycobacterial agent

Tablet – 400mg, 500mg, 750mg, 1000mg

MOA- Pyrazinamide is a prodrug which stops the growth of Mycobacterium Tuberculosis. To get the active form of pyrazinoic acid, the conversion of enzyme pyrazinamidase to pyrazinamide takes place [27]. The pH of 5 to 6 i.e. in acidic conditions, the pyrazinoic acid slowly leaks out and converts to the protonated conjugate acid. Inside the bacillus, it accumulates at the acidic pH rather than at neutral pH [27, 28].

Pyrazinoic acid was known to inhibit the enzyme Fatty Acid Synthase (FAS) I. Therefore the accumulation of pyrazinoic acid disrupts membrane potential which is necessary for the survival of M. tuberculosis at an acidic site of infection.

For pyrazinamide susceptibility, acidic environment is not essential and treatment does not lead to rapid disruption of membrane potential [29]. Pyrazinoic acid binds to the ribosomal protein S1 (RpsA) and inhibits trans-translation [30].

Pharmacokinetic Data: - The bioavailability is >90% and the metabolism occur in the liver and the biological half-life is 9 to 10hrs and excretion through kidneys.

Pregnancy Category: - C

Routes of Administration: - Oral

Dosage and Administration:-

Adults and children (for the first two or three months) – 25mg/kg daily (20-30mg/kg)

35mg/kg (30-40mg/kg) three times weekly

50mg/kg (40-60mg/kg) two times weekly

Contraindications: - Known hypersensitivity and severe hepatic impairment

Adverse Effects:-

Though hypersensitivity reactions are rare, there are some patients who complain of slight flushing of the skin. During the early phases of treatment moderate rise in serum, transaminase concentration are common. Severe hepatotoxicity is rare occurring condition due to inhibition of renal tubular secretions, a hyperuricemia occurs usually, but this is asymptomatic at most times. Arthralgia occurs commonly and is responsive to simple analgesics. With intermittent administration of pyrazinamide, both hyperuricemia and arthralgia may be reduced. Pyrazinamide is the common cause of drug-induced hepatitis among the standard four-drug regimen isoniazid, rifampicin, pyrazinamide, and ethambutol [31].

Over Dosage:-

Little had been recorded on the management of pyrazinamide overdose. Acute liver damage and hyperuricemia have been reported. Treatment is essentially symptomatic. Emesis and gastric lavage can be done if undertaken within a few hours of ingestion. There is no specific antidote, treatment is supportive.

Storage:-

Tablets should be stored in tightly closed containers and protected from light.

11. Ethambutol

Group- Anti mycobacterial agent

Tablet – 400mg (hydrochloride), 600mg, 800mg, 1000mg, 1200mg

Moa- It acts by the obstruction of cell wall formation. By the attachment of mycolic acids to residues of arabinogalactan, it forms a mycolyl-arabinogalactan-peptidoglycan complex in the cell wall. By inhibition of enzyme arabinosyl transferase, it disrupts arabinogalactan synthesis. By this it leads to increased permeability of the cell wall.

Pharmacokinetic Data – It is readily absorbed from the gastrointestinal tract. Plasma concentration peak achieves in two to four hours and decay with a half-life of three to four hours. It is excreted in the urine both unchanged and as inactive hepatic metabolites. About 20% is excreted in the feces as unchanged drug.

Pregnancy Category – C

Routes of Administration – Oral

Dosage and Administration –

Adults – 15mg/kg (15-20mg/kg) daily

30mg/kg (25-35mg/kg) three times weekly, or

45mg/kg (40-50mg/kg) two times weekly

Children – max 15mg/kg daily

Contraindications – Known hypersensitivity, Pre-existing optic neuritis from any cause, Inability (for example due to young age) to report symptomatic visual disturbances and Creatinine clearance of less than 50ml/min.

Side Effects - Common side effects are joint pain, nausea, headaches, and feeling tired [32]. Liver problems and allergic reactions may also occur [32].

Adverse Effects – Dose-dependent optic neuritis can readily result in impairment of visual acuity and color vision. Blindness can occur if treatment is not discontinued promptly, but early changes are usually reversible. Signs of peripheral neuritis occasionally develop in the legs

Over Dosage – Emesis and gastric lavage can be done if undertaken within a few hours of ingestion. Subsequently, dialysis may be of value. Treatment is supportive and there is no specific antidote.

Storage – Tablets should be stored in well-closed containers

12. Streptomycin

Group – Aminoglycoside antibiotic

MOA - Streptomycin is a protein synthesis inhibitor. Streptomycin binds to 16S rRNA of 30S subunit by interfering with intermediate binding to 30S subunit [33]. This leads to inhibition of protein synthesis and ultimately death of microbial cells. In association with mRNA strand, the binding of the molecule to the 30S subunit interferes with 50S subunit. This reveals an unstable ribosomal-mRNA complex, which leads to a frameshift and defective protein synthesis, which finally results in cell death [34]. The ribosome's present in humans is structurally different from those in bacteria, so the drug doesn't have any effect in human cells. It inhibits both Gram-positive and Gram-negative bacteria [35] and is useful as a broad-spectrum antibiotic.

Pharmacokinetic Data – It is not absorbed from gastrointestinal tract but, after intramuscular administration, it diffuses readily into the extracellular component of most body tissues. The half-life of plasma is normally for up to two to three hours and it is considerably extended in the new-born, in the elderly and in patients with severe renal impairment. It is excreted unchanged in the urine.

Pregnancy Category – D

Routes of Administration – IM, IV

Dosage and Administration –

Adults and children – 15mg/kg (12-18mg/kg) daily, or two or three times weekly

Contraindications – Known hypersensitivity, Auditory nerve impairment and Myasthenia gravis

Side Effects - Common side effects are vomiting, numbness of the face, fever, and rash [36].

Adverse Effects –

Vestibular function impairment is not common with currently recommended doses. Dosage should decrease if vertigo, headache, vomiting, and tinnitus occur.

Compared to other aminoglycosides antibiotics streptomycin is less nephrotoxic. If urinary output falls or albuminuria occurs or tubular casts are detected then dosage must be reduced by half immediately.

Drug Interactions –

The patients who receive streptomycin, other ototoxic or nephrotoxic drugs should not be administered. These include other aminoglycosides antibiotics, amphotericin B, cephalosporins, ethacrynic acid, cyclosporine, cisplatin, furosemide, and vancomycin

Over Dosage – Hemodialysis can be beneficial. There is no specific antidote and treatment is supportive.

Storage –

Solutions retain their potency for 48 hours after reconstitution at room temp and for up to 14 days when refrigerated. Powder for injection should be stored in lightly closed containers protected from light.

References

1. Dolin, Gerald L Mandell, John E et al. Mandell, Douglas, and Bennett's principles and practice of infectious diseases. Philadelphia, PA. 2010, 7th edition, Churchill Livingstone-Elsevier. Chapter 250.
2. https://goo.gl/images/h2KPG7
3. World Health Organization (WHO) Global Tuberculosis Report 2013. Geneva: 2013.
4. https://www.ncbi.nlm.nih.gov/pmc/articles/PMC4235436/figure/f1-mjhid-6-1-e2014070/
5. Crowley, Leonard V. An introduction to human disease: pathology and pathophysiology correlations. Sudbury, Mass. 2010, 8th edition. Jones and Bartlett. p. 374
6. World Health Organization (2011). The sixteenth global report on tuberculosis. Archived from the original (PDF) on 6 September 2012.
7. ATS/CDC Statement committee on Latent Tuberculosis Infection.Targeted tuberculin testing and treatment of latent tuberculosis infection. American Thoracic Society"2000. MMWR Recommendations and Reports. 49: p.1-51.
8. van Zyl Smit RN, Pai M, Yew WW, et al. Global lung health: the colliding epidemics of tuberculosis, tobacco smoking, HIV and COPD. European Respiratory Journal. 2010, 35 (1): 27–33.
9. Ahmed N, Hasnain S. Molecular epidemiology of tuberculosis in India: Moving forward with a systems biology approach". Tuberculosis. 2011. 91 (5): 407-3
10. https://goo.gl/images/49ULYm
11. Lawn SD, Zumla AI. Tuberculosis. Lancet. 2011, 378 (9785): 57–72.
12. Behera, D. Textbook of Pulmonary Medicine (2nd ed.). New Delhi: Jaypee Brothers Medical Publishers. 2010 p. 457. ISBN 978-81-8448-749-7. Archived from the original on 6 September 2015.
13. Jindal, editor-in-chief SK. Textbook of Pulmonary and Critical Care Medicine. New Delhi: Jaypee Brothers Medical Publishers. 2011. p. 549. ISBN 978-93-5025-073-0. Archived from the original on 7 September 2015
14. Golden MP, Vikram HR. Extrapulmonary tuberculosis: an overview. American Family Physician. 2005.72 (9): 1761-1768

15. Dolin Gerald L Mandell, John E Bennett, Raphael. Mandell, Douglas, and Bennett's principles and practice of infectious diseases (7th ed.). Philadelphia, PA:2010, 7th edition. Churchill Livingstone/Elsevier. pp. Chapter 250

16. Ghosh, Thomas M Habermann, Amit K. Mayo Clinic internal medicine: concise textbook. Rochester, MN: Mayo Clinic Scientific Press. 2008. p. 789. ISBN 978-1-4200-6749-1.

17. Escalante. In the clinic. Tuberculosis. Annals of Internal Medicine. 2009, 150 (11):2.

18. Bento J Silva As, Rodrigue F, Duarte R. Diagnostic tools in tuberculosis. Acta Medica Porguesa. 2011, 24(1):145-154.

19. Kumar V, Abbas Ak, Fausto N, Mitchell RN. Robbins Basic Pathology. Saunders Elsevier, 8th edition: 516-522.

20. Lawn SD, Zumla AI. Tuberculosis. Lancet. 2011, 378(9785):57-72

21. Roy A, Eisenunt M, Harris RJ, et al. Effect of BCG vaccination against Mycobacterium tuberculosis infection in children: systematic review and meta-analysis. BMJ. 349.

22. http://apps.who.int/iris/bitstream/10665/44165/1/9789241547833_eng.pdf?ua=1&ua=1

23. Isoniazid Suarez J, Rangauelova K, Jarzecki AA, et al. An oxyferrous heme/protein-based radical intermediate is catalytically competent in the catalase reaction of Mycobacterium tuberculosis catalase-peroxidase (KatG). The Journal of Biological Chemistry. 2009, 284(11):7017-7029.

24. https://en.wikipedia.org/wiki/Isoniazid#/media/File:Activation_of_isoniazid_with_NAD.jp

25. Rifampicin Calvori C, Frontalis L, Leoni L, Tecce G. Effect of rifampycin on protein synthesis. Nature. 1965, 207(995):417-418.

26. Rifampicin. The American Society of Health-System Pharmacists. 2015

27. Whitfield Michael G, Soeters Heidi M, Warren Robin M. York et al. A Global Perspective on Pyrazinamide Resistance: Systematic Review and Meta-Analysis. 2015. ISSN 1932-6203.

28. Zhang Y, Mitchison D. The curious characteristics of pyrazinamide: a review. Int. J. Tuberc. Lung Dis. 2003. 7 (1): 6-21.

29. Peterson Nicholas D, Rosen Brandon R, Dillon Nicholas A, et al. Uncoupling Environmental pH and Intrabacterial Acidification from Pyrazinamide Susceptibility in Mycobacterium tuberculosis. Antimicrobial Agents and Chemotherapy.2015, 59 (12): 7320-7326.

30. Shi W, Zhang X, Jiang X et al. Pyrazinamide inhibits trans-translation in Mycobacterium tuberculosis. Science. 2011, 333 (6049): 1630-1632.

31. Yee D, et al. Incidence of serious side effects from first-line antituberculosis drugs among patients treated for active tuberculosis. Am J Respir Crit Care Med. 2003, 167 (11): 1472–1477.

32. Ethambutol Hydrochloride. The American Society of Health-System Pharmacists. 2016.

33. Sharma D, Cukras AR, Rogers EJ, et al. Mutational analysis of S12 protein and implications for the accuracy of decoding by the ribosome. Journal of Molecular Biology. 2007, 374 (4): 1065-1076.

34. Raymon, Lionel P. COMLEX Level 1 Pharmacology Lecture Notes. Miami, FL: Kaplan, Inc. 2011. p. 181.

35. Jan-Thorsten Schantz, Kee-Woei Ng. A manual for primary human cell culture. World Scientific. 2004. p. 89.

36. Streptomycin Sulfate. The American Society of Health-System Pharmacists. 2016.

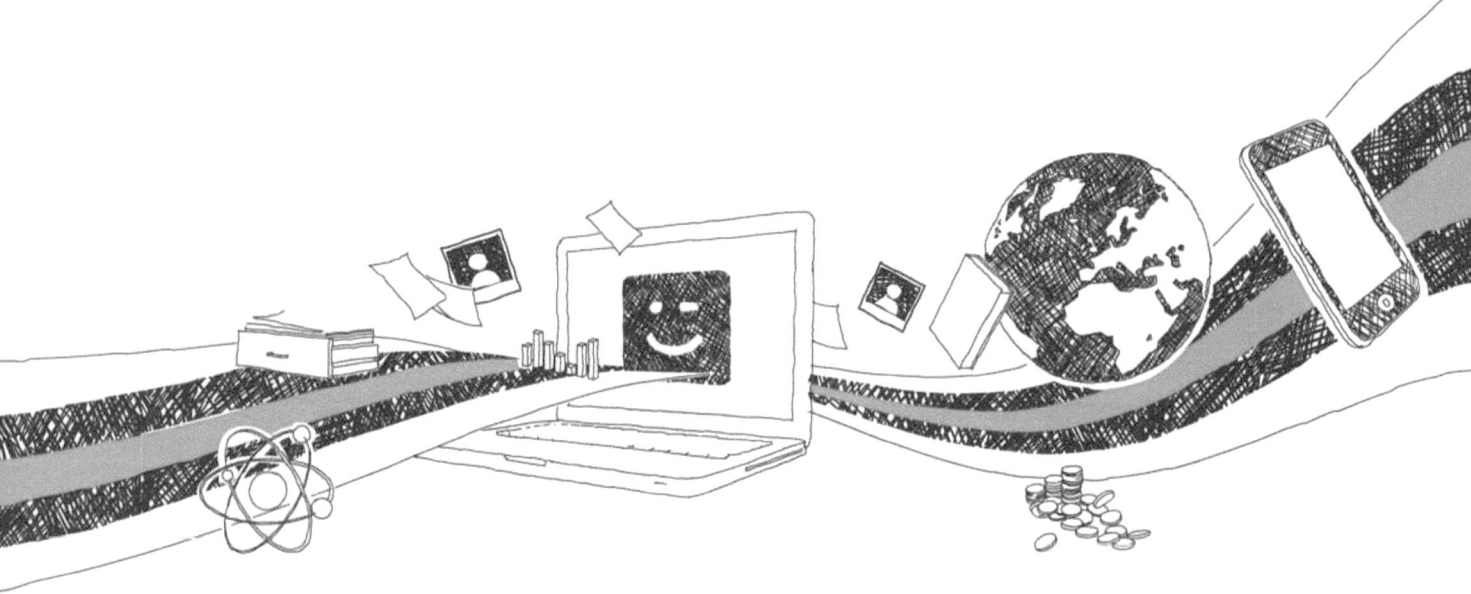
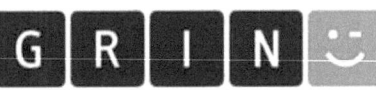